The Old Cocoon

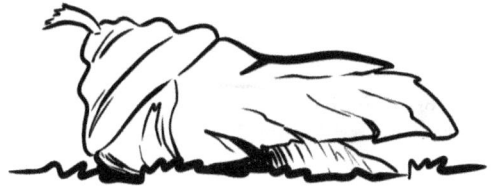

APRIL O'LEARY

Illustrated By Jonathan Rambinintsoa

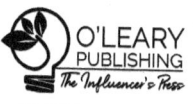

BONITA SPRINGS, FL

Copyright © 2020 by April O'Leary

All rights reserved.

Published in the United States by
O'Leary Publishing
www.olearypublishing.com

ISBN: 978-1-952491-04-7 (print)
ISBN: 978-1-952491-05-4 (ebook)
Library of Congress Control Number: 2020909191

Editing by Heather Davis Desrocher
Illustrations by Jonathan Rambinintsoa
Book Design by Jessica Angerstein

This Book Belongs To

With Love From

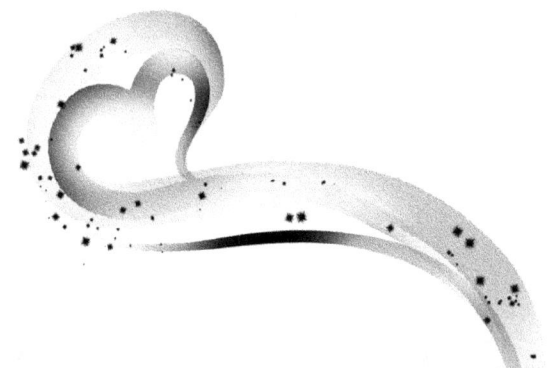

We delight in the
beauty of the butterfly,
but rarely admit
the changes it has gone through
to achieve that beauty.

—Maya Angelou

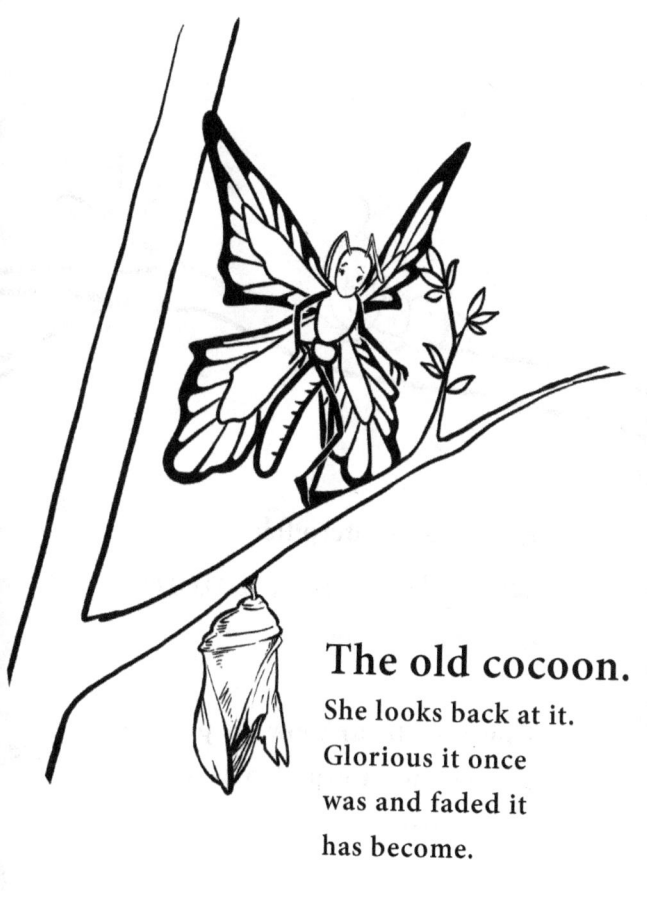

The old cocoon.

She looks back at it.
Glorious it once
was and faded it
has become.

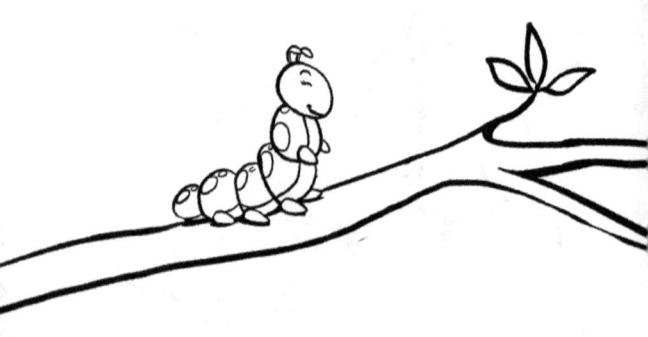

Her life as a caterpillar
was pleasant enough,
or so she thought.

How was she to know the process?
She had never experienced a
metamorphosis before.

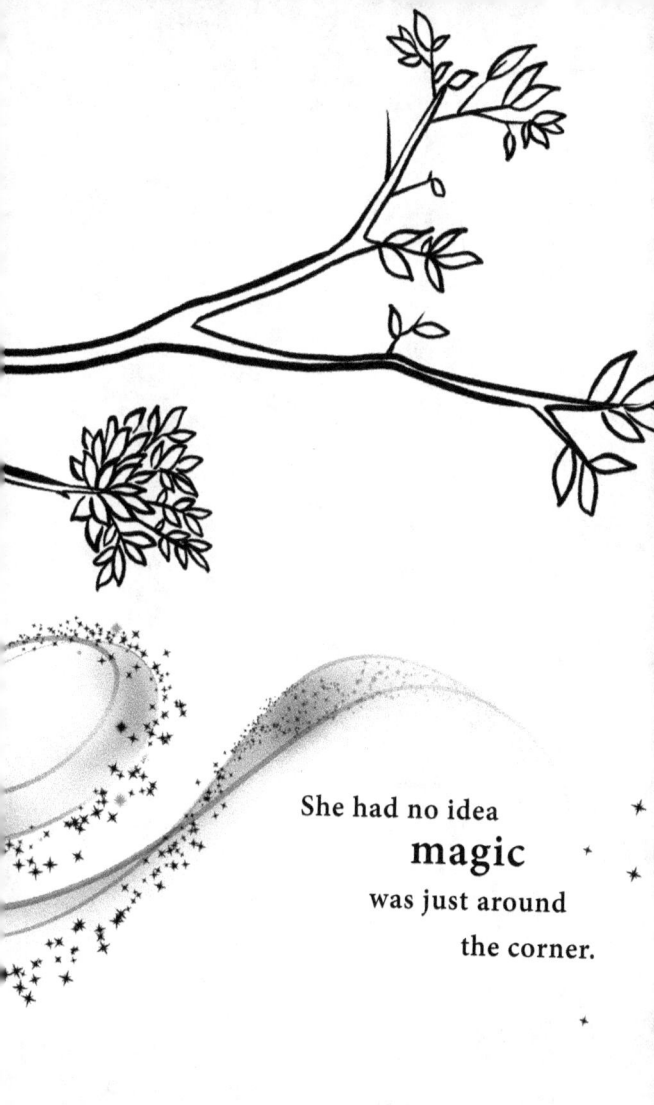

She had no idea **magic** was just around the corner.

One night, after filling up on all the good in life, the caterpillar spun herself into darkness.

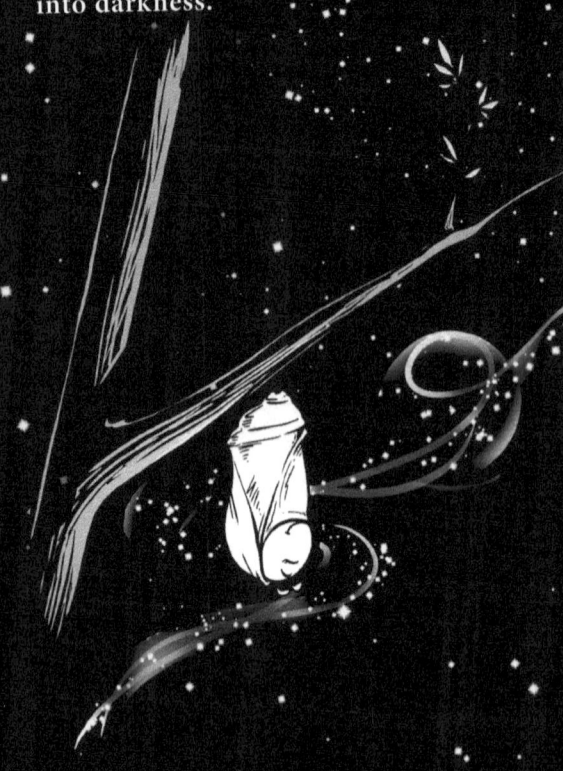

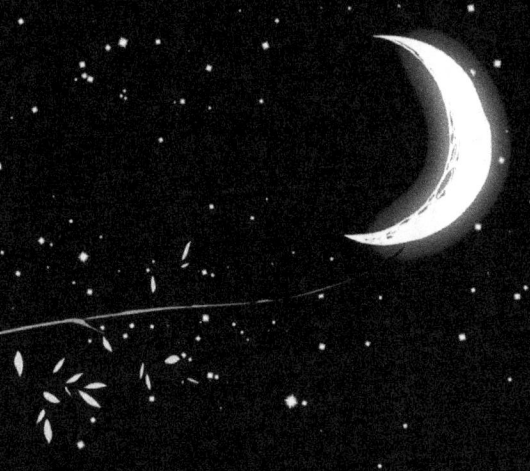

The light of day faded and a deep sleep came over her. The subtle pain of change came in waves, rising and falling, over and over again.

What was happening?

The security and oneness she experienced with the cocoon were like nothing she had known in her life.

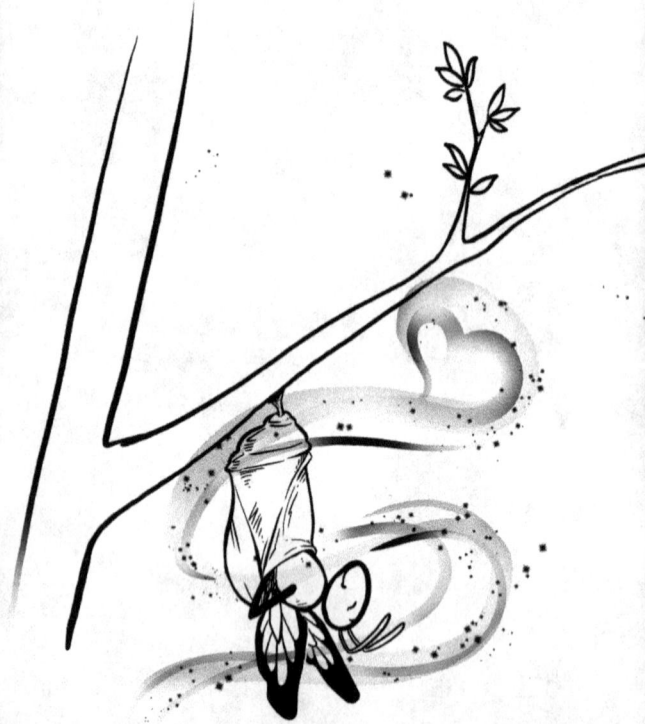

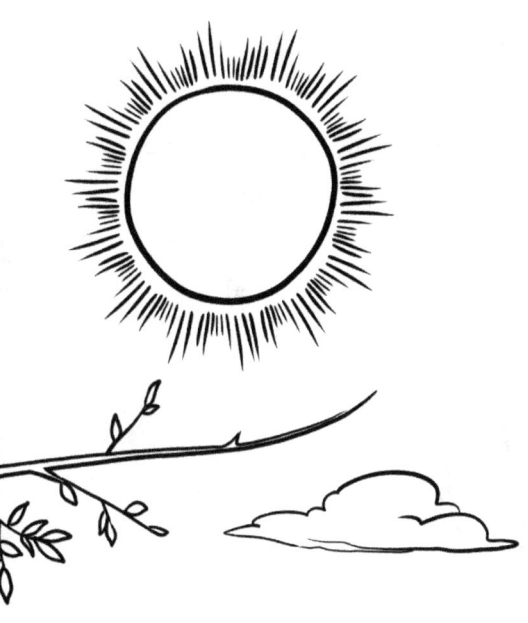

Then the fateful day arrived when their time together was complete. The cocoon slowly broke open and

gently let her go.

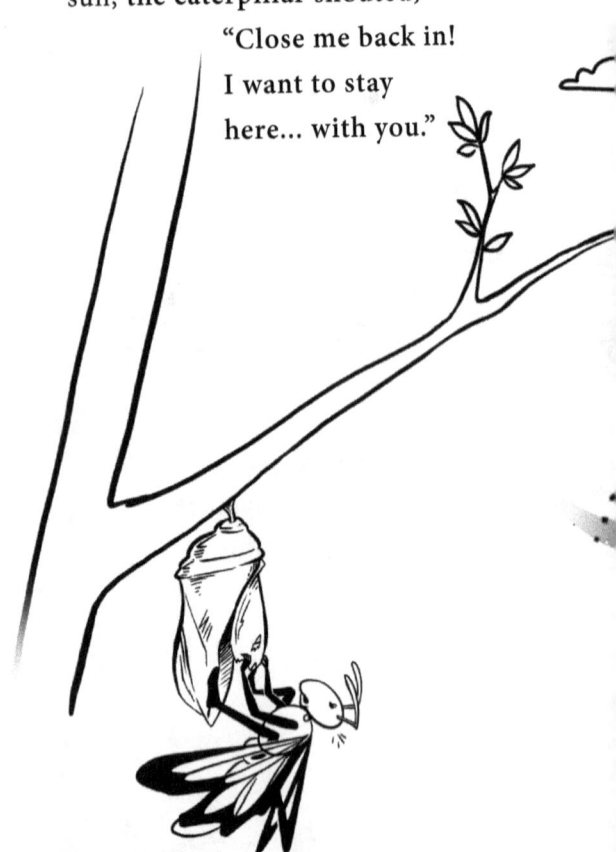

Awakened by the light of the sun, the caterpillar shouted, "Close me back in! I want to stay here... with you."

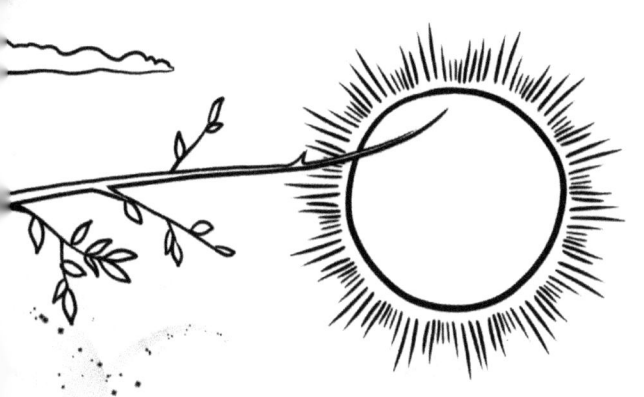

In awe of her beauty,
the cocoon softly replied,
"Look! You have changed.
We have loved each other well,
but now it is time for you to
**spread your wings
and FLY.**"

Sadness swept over the butterfly. Their sweet season together had come to an end.

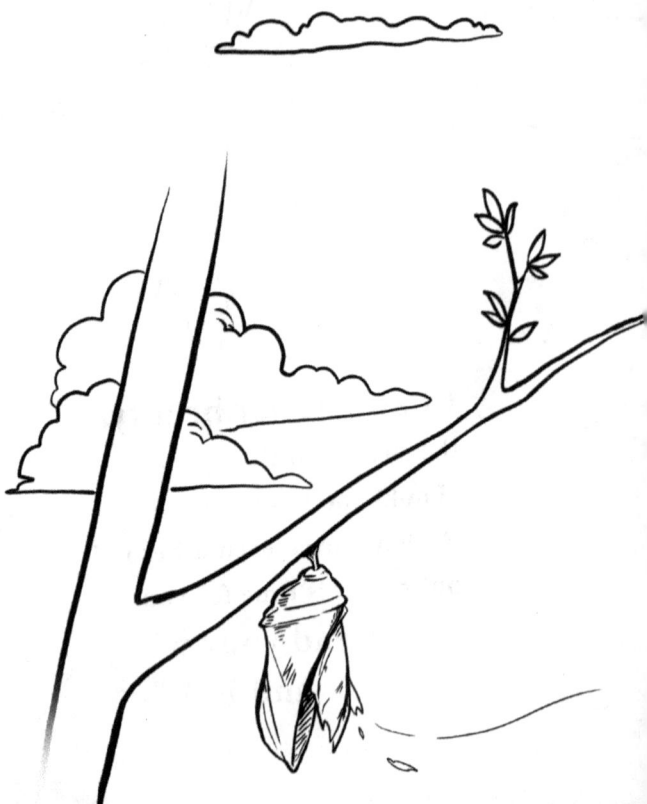

Sitting alone, as the hours passed, a new pain settled in. The pain of separation was even greater than the **pain of change.**

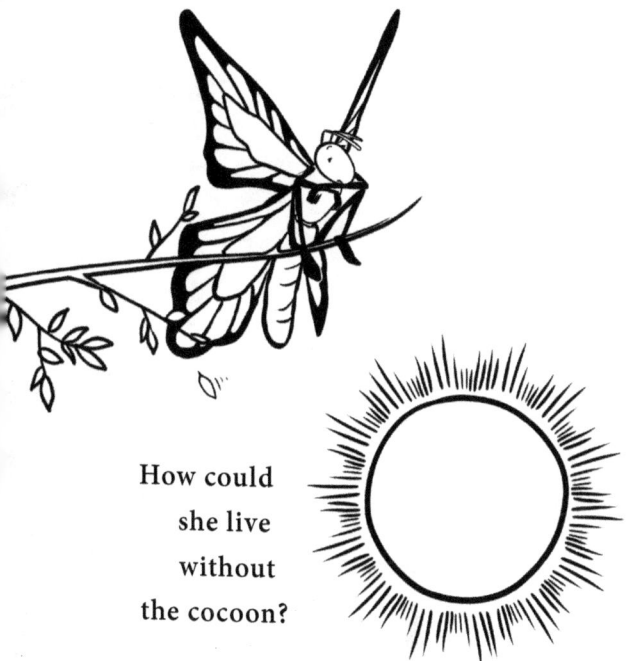

How could she live without the cocoon?

Slowly a tingling warmth of **acceptance** rose up from within her.

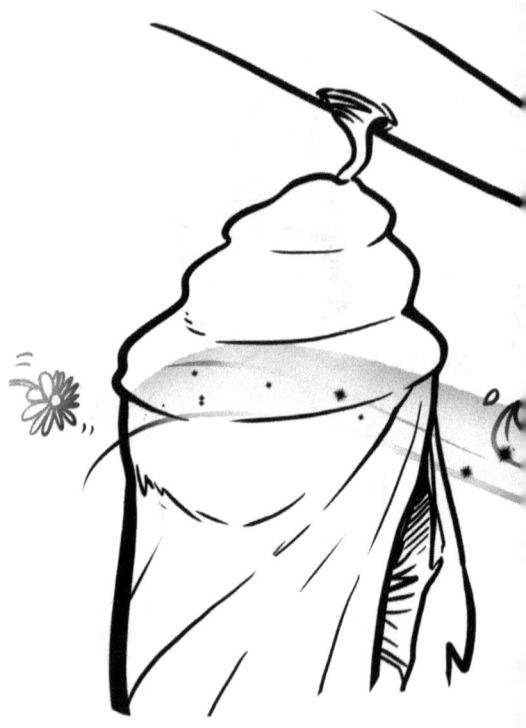

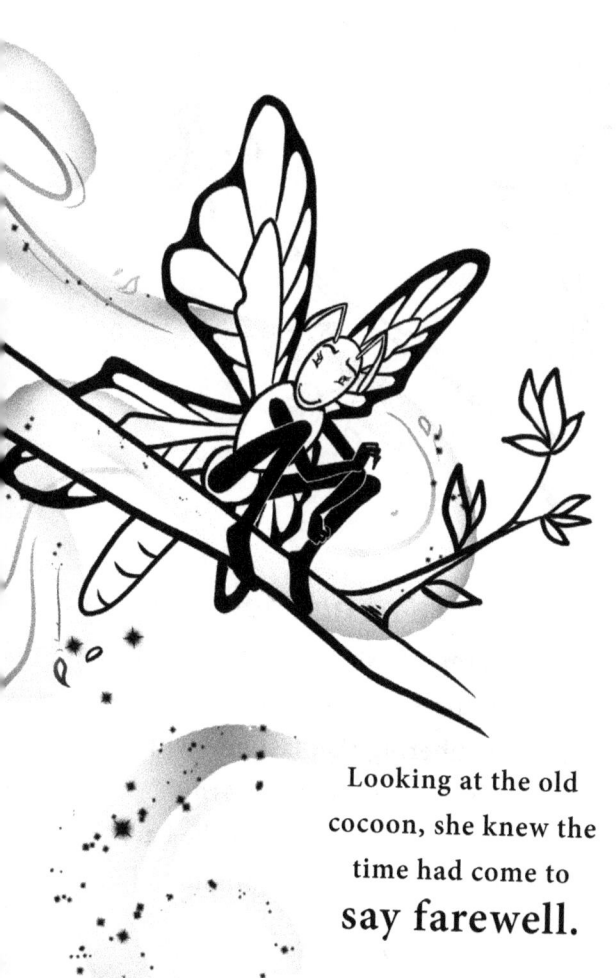

Looking at the old cocoon, she knew the time had come to **say farewell.**

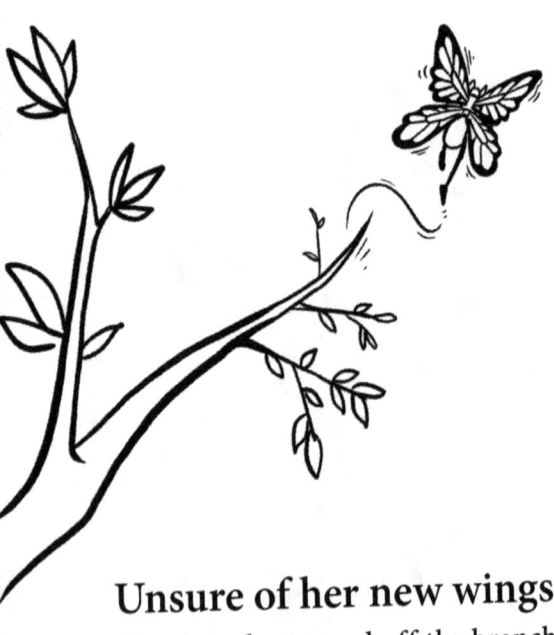

Unsure of her new wings,
she gingerly stepped off the branch
and flitted away carefully,
remembering that last moment
when the old cocoon's warmth
still surrounded her and she had
not yet taken her first flight.

Although the days passed, and the **butterfly grew stronger,** life often became hard. She sometimes wished she could transform back into a caterpillar.

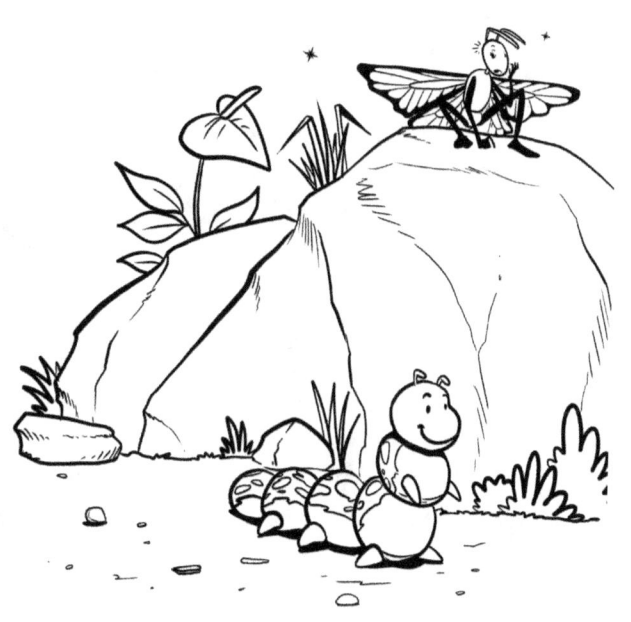

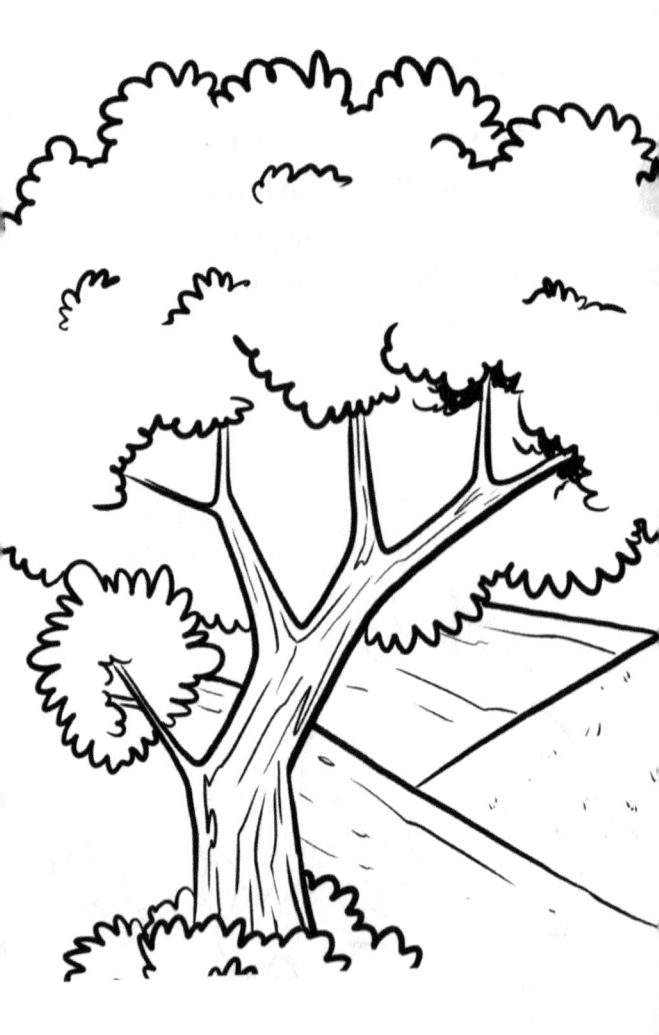

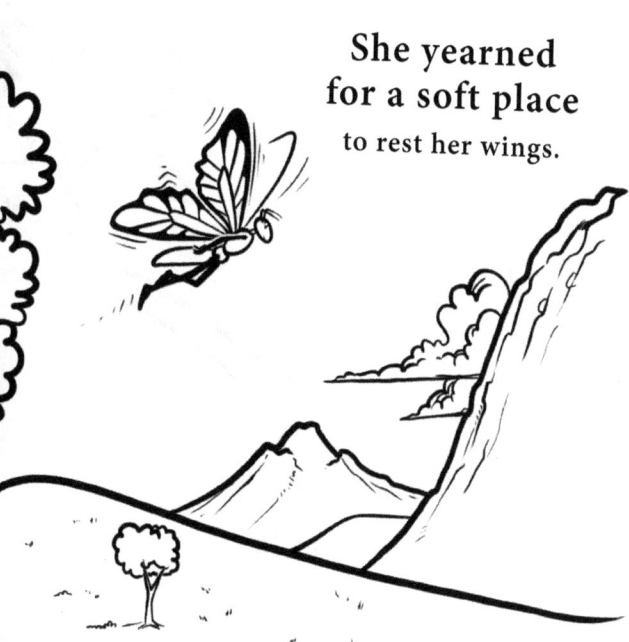

She yearned for a soft place to rest her wings.

She missed the **security, comfort, and ease** the old cocoon had given her.

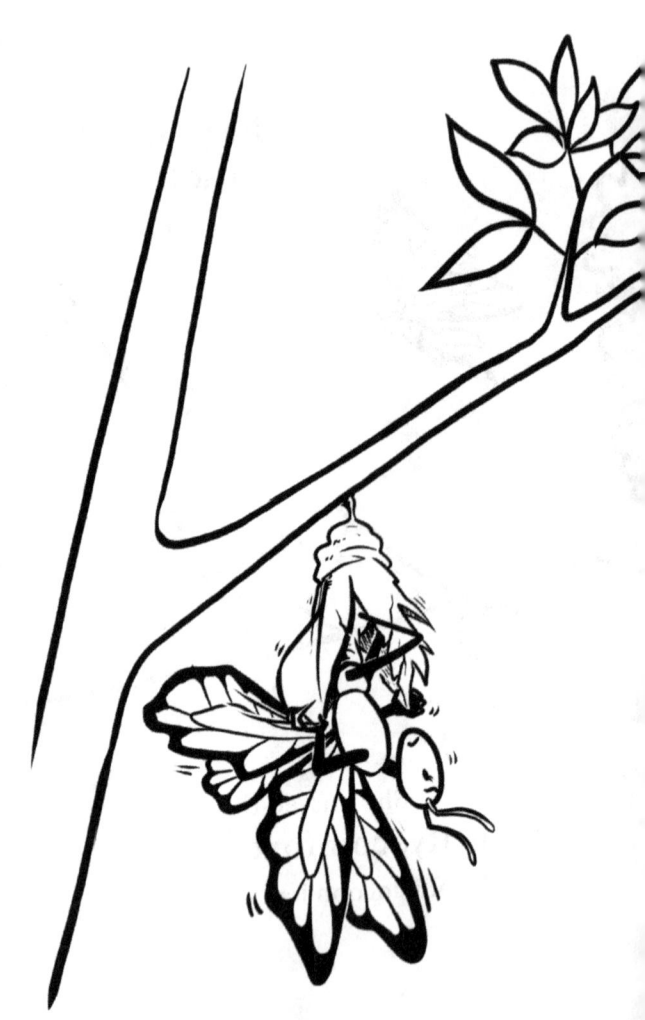

Once she secretly visited that place she used to call home.

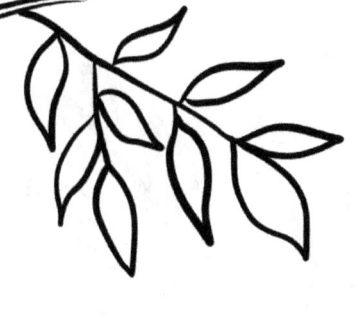

She desperately tried to fit in...
Squeezing.
Tucking.
Remembering.
Could the old cocoon have its own metamorphosis too?
she wondered.

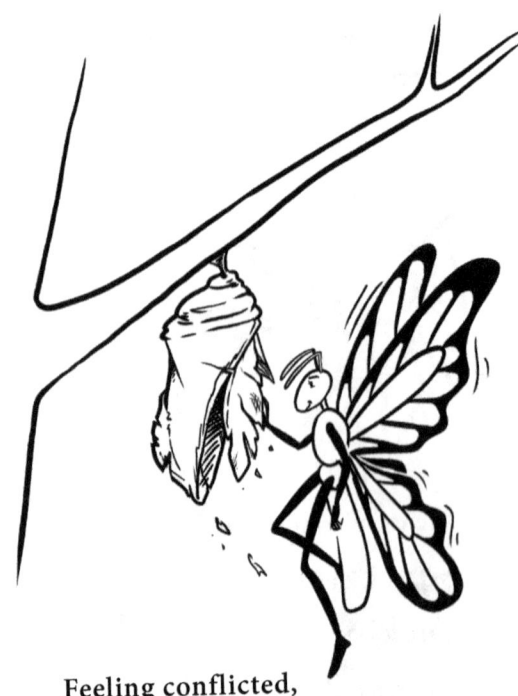

Feeling conflicted,
yet strangely confident her plan might work,
she began refashioning the old cocoon.

Coloring and painting.
Cutting and pasting.
This life, she thought,
is short and full of mystery.

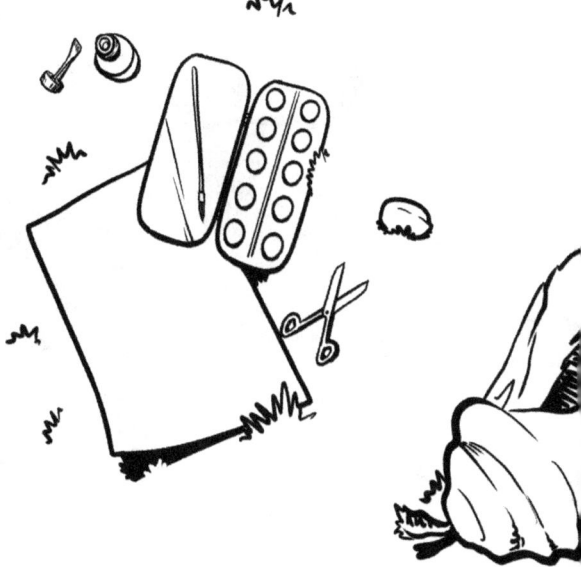

She smiled as she admired her work.

Suddenly she realized
that the old cocoon lived on,

**not only in her art,
but in her heart.**

The magic she experienced
was inside of her all along.

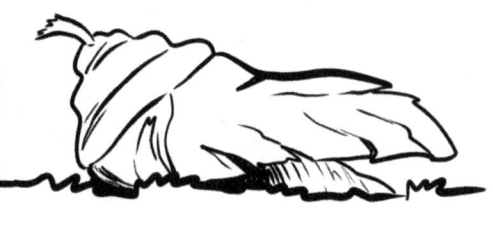

The old cocoon
simply helped her to
believe in herself.

She has heard of ones like her
**who have changed
the atmosphere**
thousands of miles away, with the
simple movement of their wings.

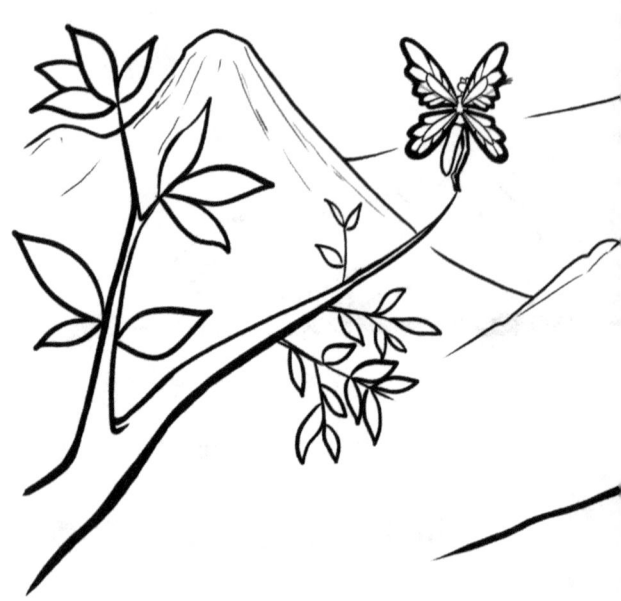

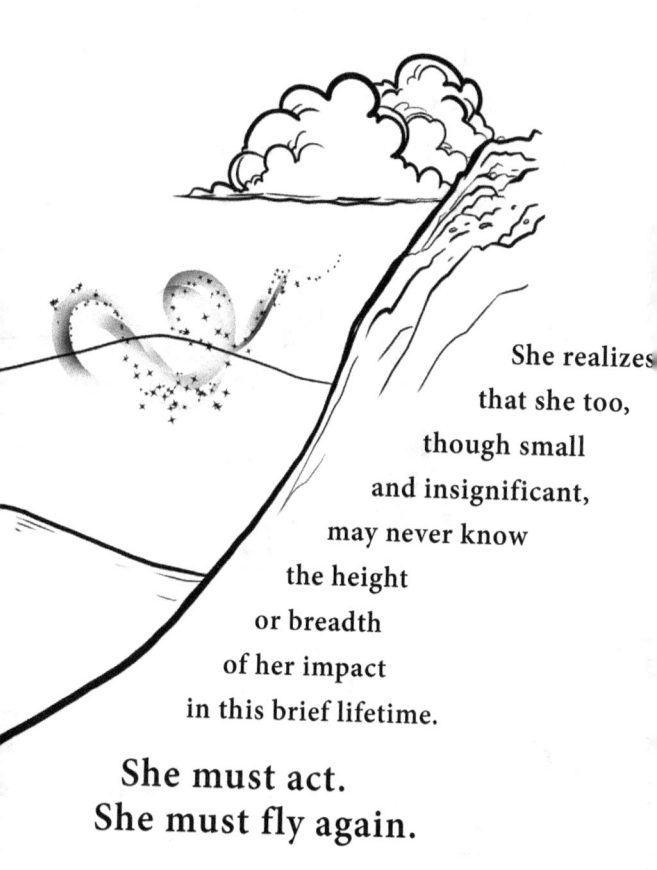

She realizes
that she too,
though small
and insignificant,
may never know
the height
or breadth
of her impact
in this brief lifetime.

**She must act.
She must fly again.**

Taking a giant leap off the branch she confidently flies into the sunset holding old cocoon in her heart.

They are one again, as they always were.

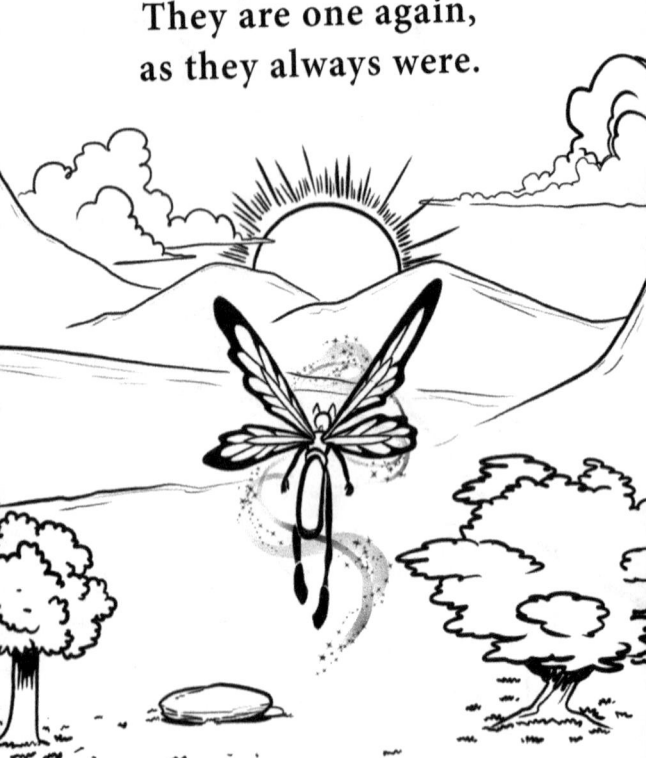

The butterfly and the old cocoon.

Follow me...

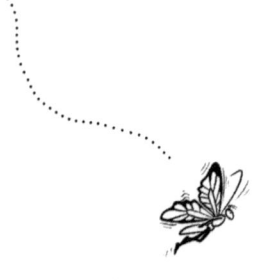

Love this book? Place a bulk order and help us spread the joy of transition and transformation with your friends and family.

Retail store? We'd love to hear from you too. Simple countertop display available for your customers to purchase *The Old Cocoon* at check out.

Visit www.olearypublishing.com/oldcocoon for wholesale pricing and direct shipping.

CPSIA information can be obtained
at www.ICGtesting.com
Printed in the USA
LVHW021546310720
662076LV00019B/716